Keto Diet Cookbook for Weight Loss 2021

Quick, Tasty and Healthy Everyday Ketogenic Recipes for Beginners

Juliana Diaz

© Copyright 2021 - Juliana Diaz - All rights reserved.

The content contained within this book may not be reproduced, duplicated or transmitted without direct written permission from the author or the publisher.

Under no circumstances will any blame or legal responsibility be held against the publisher, or author, for any damages, reparation, or monetary loss due to the information contained within this book. Either directly or indirectly.

Legal Notice:

This book is copyright protected. This book is only for personal use. You cannot amend, distribute, sell, use, quote or paraphrase any part, or the content within this book, without the consent of the author or publisher.

Disclaimer Notice:

Please note the information contained within this document is for educational and entertainment purposes only. All effort has been executed to present accurate, up to date, and reliable, complete information. No warranties of any kind are declared or implied. Readers acknowledge that the author is not engaging in the rendering of legal, financial, medical or professional advice. The content within this book has been derived from various sources. Please consult a licensed professional before attempting any techniques outlined in this book.

By reading this document, the reader agrees that under no circumstances is the author responsible for any losses, direct or indirect, which are incurred as a result of the use of information contained within this document, including, but not limited to, — errors, omissions, or inaccuracies

Table of Content

- SMOOTHIES & BREAKFAST RECIPES 9
- Quick & Easy Blueberry Chaffle 10
- Apple Cinnamon Chaffles 12
- Cinnamon Cream Cheese Chaffle 14
- Choco Chip Pumpkin Chaffle 16
- Maple Chaffle 18
- Sweet Vanilla Chocolate Chaffle 20
- Mozzarella Peanut Butter Chaffle 22
- Choco Chip Lemon Chaffle 24
- Cherry Chocolate Chaffle 26
- Apple GingerBlueberry Smoothie 27
- CheeseBlueberrySmoothie 29
- Peanut Butter Sandwich Chaffle 30
- PORK, BEEF & LAMB RECIPES 32
- Pan Fry Pork Chops 33
- SEAFOOD & FISH RECIPES 34
- Buffalo Fish 34
- Buttered Scallops 36
- Garlic Shrimp 37
- Garlicky Lemon Scallops 38
- Garlic Parmesan Cod 40
- Spinach Shrimp Alfredo 42
- MEATLESS MEALS 34
- Cauliflower Broccoli Rice 35
- SOUPS, STEWS & SALADS 37
- Hearty Cabbage Beef Soup 38
- BRUNCH & DINNER 40
- Cheese Almond Pancakes 41
- BREAKFAST RECIPES 42

Cauliflower Toastwith Avocado 42
DESSERTS & DRINKS 44
Cheesecake Fat Bombs 44
APPETIZERS AND DESSERTS 46
Almond Flour Crackers 46
PORK AND BEEFRECIPES 48
Cheesy Beef 48
Keto Minced Meat 50
Keto Taco Casserole 51
SEAFOOD RECIPES 53
Mahi Mahi Stew 53
VEGAN & VEGETARIAN 55
Cauliflower Gratin 55
CHICKEN AND POULTRY RECIPES 57
Chicken Enchiladas 57
BREAKFAST RECIPES 59
Cinnamon Noatmeal 59
Almond Coconut Porridge 60
Vegetable TofuScramble 61
LUNCH RECIPES 63
Asparagus Mash 63
Classic Cabbage Slaw 65
Delicious Herb Cauliflower Rice 66
DINNER RECIPES 67
Almond Green Beans 67
Fried Okra 68
DESSERT RECIPES 69
Lemon Mousse 69
BREAKFAST RECIPES 70
Burrito Bowl 70

Burger Cabbage Stir Fry 72
UNUSUAL DELICIOUS MEAL RECIPES 74
Calamari Salad 74
KETO DESSERTS RECIPES 76
Coconut Lemon Bars 76
CAKE 78
Fudgy Chocolate Cake 78
Coconut Cake 80
Intermediate: Lemon Cake 82
Tarts and Pie: Beginner 84
Raspberry Sorbet 86
Broken Black PepperBread 88
LUNCH RECIPES 91
Herb Bread 91
Spicy Cloud Bread 93
SNACKS RECIPES 94
Sesame bread 94
Buns with sesame 95
THE KETO LUNCH 97
Tuesday:Lunch:MasonJar Salad 97
Wednesday: Lunch: The Smoked Salmon Special 99
Thursday: Dinner: On the go chicken wings with green beans 100

SMOOTHIES & BREAKFAST

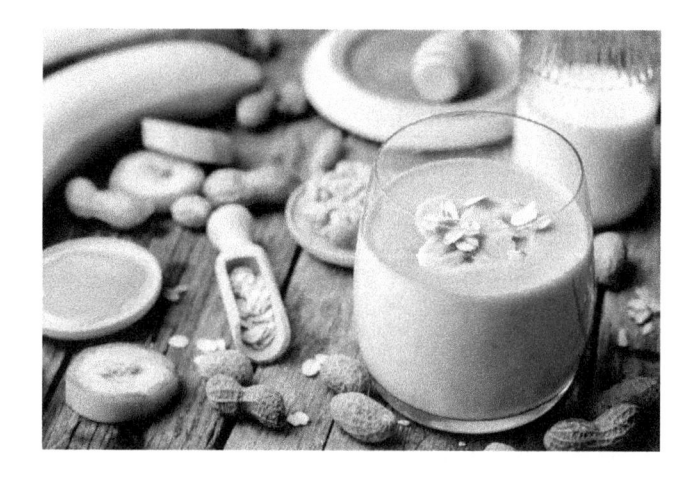

Quick & Easy Blueberry Chaffle

Preparation Time: 15 minutes

Servings: 2

Ingredients:

- 1 egg, lightly beaten
- 1/4 cup blueberries
- 1/2 tsp vanilla
- 1 oz cream cheese
- 1/4 tsp baking powder, gluten-free
- 4 tsp Swerve
- 1 tbsp coconut flour

Directions:

1. Preheat your waffle maker.
2. In a small bowl, mix coconut flour, baking powder, and Swerve until well combined.
3. Add vanilla, cream cheese, egg, and vanilla and whisk until combined.
4. Spray waffle maker with cooking spray.
5. Pour half batter in the hot waffle maker and top with 4-5 blueberries and cook for 4-5 minutes until golden brown. Repeat with the remaining batter.
6. Serve and enjoy.

Nutrition:

Calories 135

Fat 8.2 g

Carbohydrates 11 g

Sugar 2.6 g

Protein 5 g

Cholesterol 97 mg

Apple Cinnamon Chaffles

Preparation Time: 20 minutes

Servings: 3

Ingredients:

- 3 eggs, lightly beaten
- 1 cup mozzarella cheese, shredded
- ¼ cup apple, chopped
- ½ tsp monk fruit sweetener
- 1 ½ tsp cinnamon
- ¼ tsp baking powder, gluten-free
- 2 tbsp coconut flour

Directions:

1. Preheat your waffle maker.
2. Add remaining ingredients and stir until well combined.
3. Spray waffle maker with cooking spray.
4. Pour 1/3 of batter in the hot waffle maker and cook for 4 minutes or until golden brown. Repeat with the remaining batter.
5. Serve and enjoy.

Nutrition:

Calories 142   Sugar 3 g

Fat 7.4 g   Protein 9.6 g

Carbohydrates 9.7 g   Cholesterol 169 mg

Cinnamon Cream Cheese Chaffle

Preparation Time: 15 minutes

Servings: 2

Ingredients:

- 2 eggs, lightly beaten
- 1 tsp collagen
- ¼ tsp baking powder, gluten-free
- 1 tsp monk fruit sweetener
- ½ tsp cinnamon
- ¼ cup cream cheese, softened
- Pinch of salt

Directions:

1. Preheat your waffle maker.
2. Add all ingredients into the bowl and beat using hand mixer until well combined.
3. Spray waffle maker with cooking spray.
4. Pour 1/2 batter in the hot waffle maker and cook for 3-4 minutes or until golden brown. Repeat with the remaining batter.
5. Serve and enjoy.

Nutrition:

Calories 179　　　　　Sugar 0.4 g
Fat 14.5 g　　　　　　Protein 10.8 g
Carbohydrates 1.9 g　　Cholesterol 196 mg

Choco Chip Pumpkin Chaffle

Preparation Time: 15 minutes

Servings: 2

Ingredients:

- 1 egg, lightly beaten
- 1 tbsp almond flour
- 1 tbsp unsweetened chocolate chips
- 1/4 tsp pumpkin pie spice
- 2 tbsp Swerve
- 1 tbsp pumpkin puree
- 1/2 cup mozzarella cheese, shredded

Directions:

1. Preheat your waffle maker.
2. In a small bowl, mix egg and pumpkin puree.
3. Add pumpkin pie spice, Swerve, almond flour, and cheese and mix well.
4. Stir in chocolate chips.
5. Spray waffle maker with cooking spray.
6. Pour half batter in the hot waffle maker and cook for 4 minutes. Repeat with the remaining batter.
7. Serve and enjoy.

Nutrition:

Calories 130

Fat 9.2 g

Carbohydrates 5.9 g

Sugar 0.6 g

Protein 6.6 g

Cholesterol 86 mg

Maple Chaffle

Preparation Time: 15 minutes

Servings: 2

Ingredients:

- 1 egg, lightly beaten
- 2 egg whites
- 1/2 tsp maple extract
- 2 tsp Swerve
- 1/2 tsp baking powder, gluten-free
- 2 tbsp almond milk
- 2 tbsp coconut flour

Directions:

1. Preheat your waffle maker.
2. In a bowl, whip egg whites until stiff peaks form.
3. Stir in maple extract, Swerve, baking powder, almond milk, coconut flour, and egg.
4. Spray waffle maker with cooking spray.
5. Pour half batter in the hot waffle maker and cook for 3-5 minutes or until golden brown. Repeat with the remaining batter.
6. Serve and enjoy.

Nutrition:

Calories 122   Sugar 1 g
Fat 6.6 g   Protein 7.7 g
Carbohydrates 9 g   Cholesterol 82 mg

Sweet Vanilla Chocolate Chaffle

Preparation Time: 10 minutes

Servings: 1

Ingredients:

- 1 egg, lightly beaten
- 1/4 tsp cinnamon
- 1/2 tsp vanilla
- 1 tbsp Swerve
- 2 tsp unsweetened cocoa powder
- 1 tbsp coconut flour
- 2 oz cream cheese, softened

Directions:

1. Add all ingredients into the small bowl and mix until well combined.
2. Spray waffle maker with cooking spray.
3. Pour batter in the hot waffle maker and cook until golden brown.
4. Serve and enjoy.

Nutrition:

Calories 312　　　　　　　　Sugar 0.8 g
Fat 25.4 g　　　　　　　　　Protein 11.6 g
Carbohydrates 11.5 g　　　　Cholesterol 226 mg

Mozzarella Peanut Butter Chaffle

Preparation Time: 15 minutes

Servings: 2

Ingredients:

- 1 egg, lightly beaten
- 2 tbsp peanut butter
- 2 tbsp Swerve
- 1/2 cup mozzarella cheese, shredded

Directions:

1. Preheat your waffle maker.
2. In a bowl, mix egg, cheese, Swerve, and peanut butter until well combined.
3. Spray waffle maker with cooking spray.
4. Pour half batter in the hot waffle maker and cook for 4 minutes or until golden brown. Repeat with the remaining batter.
5. Serve and enjoy.

Nutrition:

Calories 150

Fat 11.5 g

Carbohydrates 5.6 g

Sugar 1.7 g

Protein 8.8 g

Cholesterol 86 mg

Choco Chip Lemon Chaffle

Preparation Time: 15 minutes

Servings: 2

Ingredients:

- 2 eggs, lightly beaten
- 1 tbsp unsweetened chocolate chips
- 2 tsp Swerve
- 1/2 tsp vanilla
- 1/2 tsp lemon extract
- 1/2 cup mozzarella cheese, shredded
- 2 tsp almond flour

Directions:

1. Preheat your waffle maker.
2. In a bowl, whisk eggs, Swerve, vanilla, lemon extract, cheese, and almond flour.
3. Add chocolate chips and stir well.
4. Spray waffle maker with cooking spray.
5. Pour 1/2 of the batter in the hot waffle maker and cook for 4-5 minutes or until golden brown. Repeat with the remaining batter.
6. Serve and enjoy.

Nutrition:

Calories 157 Sugar 0.7 g
Fat 10.8 g Protein 9 g
Carbohydrates 5.4 g Cholesterol 167 mg

Cherry Chocolate Chaffle

Preparation Time: 10 minutes
Servings: 1

Ingredients:

- 1 egg, lightly beaten
- 1 tbsp unsweetened chocolate chips
- 2 tbsp sugar-free cherry pie filling
- 2 tbsp heavy whipping cream
- 1/2 cup mozzarella cheese, shredded
- 1/2 tsp baking powder, gluten-free
- 1 tbsp Swerve
- 1 tbsp unsweetened cocoa powder
- 1 tbsp almond flour

Directions:

1. Preheat the waffle maker.
2. In a bowl, whisk together egg, cheese, baking powder, Swerve, cocoa powder, and almond flour.
3. Spray waffle maker with cooking spray.
4. Pour batter in the hot waffle maker and cook until golden brown.
5. Top with cherry pie filling, heavy whipping cream, and chocolate chips and serve.

Nutrition:
Calories 264
Fat 22 g
Carbohydrates 8.5 g
Sugar 0.5 g
Protein 12.7 g
Cholesterol 212 mg

Apple Ginger Blueberry Smoothie

Preparation Time: 5 minutes Cooking Time: 5 minutes Serve: 2

Ingredients:

- 1/2 apple
- 1 tsp MCT oil
- 1/2 tbsp collagen powder
- 1 tsp ginger
- 1 cup unsweetened coconut milk
- 1/2 cup coconut yogurt
- 15 blueberries

Directions:

1. Add all ingredients into the blender and blend until smooth.
2. Serve and enjoy.

Nutritional Value (Amount per Serving):

Calories 169

Fat 15 g

Carbohydrates 5 g

Sugar 2 g

Protein 4 g

Cholesterol 5 mg

Cheese Blueberry Smoothie

Preparation Time: 5 minutes Cooking Time: 5 minutes Serve: 1

Ingredients:

- 1 cup unsweetened almond milk
- 1/2 cup ice
- 1/4 tsp vanilla
- 5 drops liquid stevia
- 1 scoop vanilla protein powder
- 1/3 cup blueberries
- 2 oz cream cheese

Directions:

1. Add all ingredients into the blender and blend until smooth.
2. Serve and enjoy.

Nutritional Value (Amount per Serving):

Calories 380

Fat 23.5 g

Carbohydrates 6.1 g

Sugar 5.3 g

Protein 32.7 g

Cholesterol 64 mg

Peanut Butter Sandwich Chaffle

Preparation Time: 15 minutes

Servings: 1

<u>Ingredients:</u>

For chaffle:

- 1 egg, lightly beaten
- 1/2 cup mozzarella cheese, shredded
- 1/4 tsp espresso powder
- 1 tbsp unsweetened chocolate chips
- 1 tbsp Swerve
- 2 tbsp unsweetened cocoa powder

For filling:

- 1 tbsp butter, softened
- 2 tbsp Swerve
- 3 tbsp creamy peanut butter

<u>Directions:</u>

1. Preheat your waffle maker.
2. In a bowl, whisk together egg, espresso powder, chocolate chips, Swerve, and cocoa powder.
3. Add mozzarella cheese and stir well.
4. Spray waffle maker with cooking spray.

5. Pour 1/2 of the batter in the hot waffle maker and cook for 3-4 minutes or until golden brown. Repeat with the remaining batter.
6. For filling: In a small bowl, stir together butter, Swerve, and peanut butter until smooth.
7. Once chaffles is cool, then spread filling mixture between two chaffle and place in the fridge for 10 minutes.
8. Cut chaffle sandwich in half and serve.

Nutrition:

Calories 190

Fat 16.1 g

Carbohydrates 9.6 g

Sugar 1.1 g

Protein 8.2 g

Cholesterol 101 mg

PORK, BEEF & LAMB RECIPES

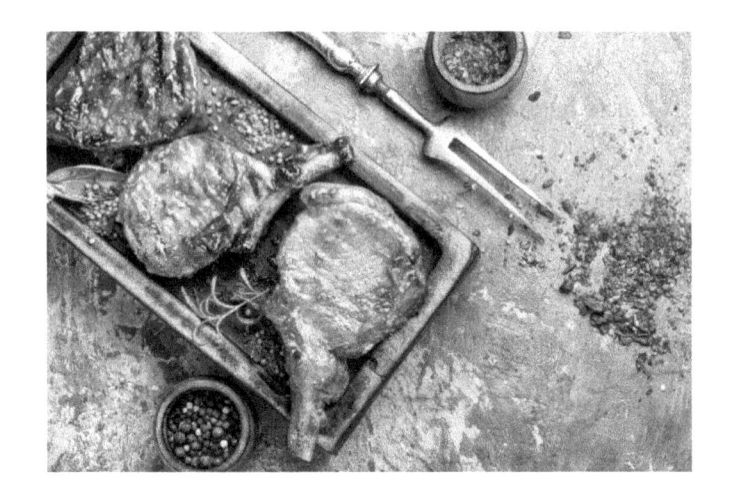

Pan Fry Pork Chops

Preparation Time: 10 minutes Cooking Time: 8 minutes

Serve: 4

Ingredients:

- 4 pork chops, boneless
- 2 tbsp olive oil
- 1/4 tsp onion powder
- 1/4 tsp garlic powder
- 1/4 tsp pepper
- Salt

Directions:

Heat oil in cast iron skillet over high heat.

1. Season pork chops with garlic powder, onion powder, pepper, and salt.
2. Sear pork chops in hot oil about 3-4 minutes on each side.
3. Serve and enjoy.

Nutritional Value (Amount per Serving):

Calories 317
Fat 26 g
Carbohydrates 0.3 g
Sugar 0.1 g
Protein 18 g
Cholesterol 69 mg

SEAFOOD & FISH RECIPES

Buffalo Fish

Serves: 3

Prep Time: 20 mins

Ingredients

- 3 tablespoons butter
- 1/3 cup Franks Red Hot sauce
- 3 fish fillets
- Salt and black pepper, to taste
- 1 teaspoon garlic powder

Directions

1. Heat butter in a large skillet and add fish fillets.
2. Cook for about 2 minutes on each side and add salt, black pepper and garlic powder.
3. Cook for about 1 minute and add Franks Red Hot sauce.
4. Cover with lid and cook for about 6 minutes on low heat.
5. Dish out on a serving platter and serve hot.

Nutrition Amount per serving

Calories 342

Total Fat 22.5g 29% Saturated Fat 8.9g 44% Cholesterol 109mg 36%

Sodium 254mg 11%

Total Carbohydrate 0.9g 0%

Dietary Fiber 0.1g 0%

Total Sugars 0.2g

Protein 34.8g

Buttered Scallops

Serves: 6

Prep Time: 15 mins

Ingredients

- 4 tablespoons fresh rosemary, chopped
- 4 garlic cloves, minced
- 2 pounds sea scallops
- Salt and black pepper, to taste
- ½ cup butter

Directions

1. Season the sea scallops with salt and black pepper.
2. Put butter, rosemary and garlic on medium high heat in a skillet.
3. Sauté for about 2 minutes and stir in the seasoned sea scallops.
4. Cook for about 3 minutes per side and dish out to serve hot.

Nutrition Amount per serving

Calories   279   Total Fat 16.8g 22%

Saturated Fat 10g 50% Cholesterol 91mg 30%

Sodium 354mg 15%

Total Carbohydrate 5.7g 2%

Dietary Fiber 1g 4% Total Sugars 0g Protein 25.8g

Garlic Shrimp

Preparation Time: 5 minutes Cooking Time: 15 minutes

Serve: 4

Ingredients:

- 1 lb shrimp, peeled and deveined
- 1 tsp parsley, chopped
- 2 tbsp lemon juice
- 5 garlic cloves, minced
- 3 tbsp butter
- Salt

Directions:

1. Melt butter in a pan over high heat.
2. Add shrimp in pan and cook for 1 minutes. Season with salt.
3. Stir and cook shrimp until turn to pink.
4. Add lemon juice and garlic and cook for 2 minutes.
5. Turn heat to medium and cook for 4 minutes more.
6. Garnish with parsley and serve.

Nutritional Value (Amount per Serving):

Calories 219

Fat 10.6 g

Carbohydrates 3.2 g

Sugar 0.2 g

Garlicky Lemon Scallops

Serves: 6

Prep Time: 30 mins

Ingredients

- 2 pounds scallops
- 3 garlic cloves, minced
- 5 tablespoons butter, divided
- Red pepper flakes, kosher salt and black pepper
- 1 lemon, zest and juice

Directions

6. Heat 2 tablespoons butter over medium heat in a large skillet and add scallops, kosher salt and black pepper.
7. Cook for about 5 minutes per side until golden and transfer to a plate.
8. Heat remaining butter in a skillet and add garlic and red pepper flakes.
9. Cook for about 1 minute and stir in lemon juice and zest
10. Return the scallops to the skillet and stir well.
11. Dish out on a platter and serve hot..

Nutrition Amount per serving

Calories 224

Total Fat 10.8g 14% Saturated Fat 6.2g 31% Cholesterol 75mg 25%

Sodium 312mg 14% Total

Carbohydrate 5.2g 2% Dietary Fiber 0.4g 1%

Total Sugars 0.3g

Protein 25.7g

Garlic Parmesan Cod

Serves: 6

Prep Time: 35 mins Ingredients

- 1 tablespoon extra-virgin olive oil
- 1 (2½) pound cod fillet
- ¼ cup parmesan cheese, finely grated
- Salt and black pepper, to taste
- 5 garlic cloves, minced

Directions

1. Preheat the oven to 4000F and grease a baking dish with cooking spray.
2. Mix together olive oil, garlic, parmesan cheese, salt and black pepper in a bowl.
3. Marinate the cod fillets in this mixture for about 1 hour.
4. Transfer to the baking dish and cover with foil.
5. Place in the oven and bake for about 20 minutes.
6. Remove from the oven and serve warm.

Nutrition Amount per serving

Calories 139 Total Fat 8g 10%

Saturated Fat 1.7g 8%

Cholesterol 37mg 12%

Sodium 77mg 3%

Total Carbohydrate 1g 0%

Dietary Fiber 0.1g 0% Total Sugars 0g

Protein 16.3g

Spinach Shrimp Alfredo

Preparation Time: 10 minutes Cooking Time: 15 minutes

Serve: 2

Ingredients:

- 1/2 lb shrimp, deveined
- 2 garlic cloves, minced
- 2 tbsp onion, chopped
- 1 cup fresh spinach, chopped
- 1/2 cup heavy cream
- 1 tbsp butter
- Pepper
- Salt

Directions:

1. Melt butter in a pan over medium heat.
2. Add onion, garlic and shrimp in the pan and sauté for 3 minutes.
3. Add remaining ingredients and simmer for 7 minutes or until cooked.
4. Serve and enjoy.

Nutritional Value (Amount per Serving):

Calories 300

Fat 19 g

Carbohydrates 5 g

Sugar 0.5 g

Protein 27 g

Cholesterol 295 mg

MEATLESS MEALS

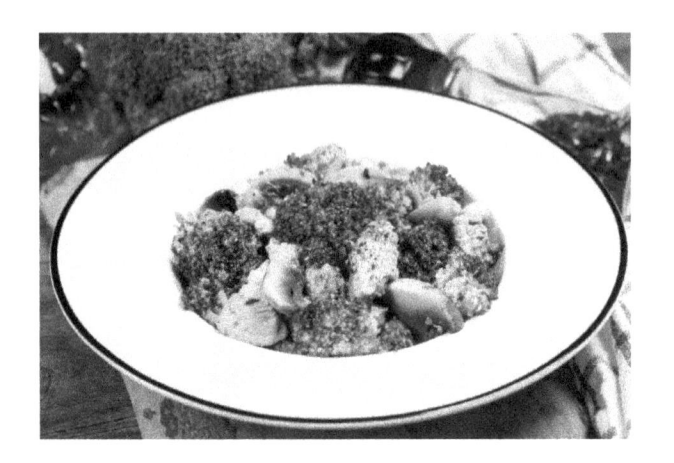

Cauliflower Broccoli Rice

Preparation Time: 10 minutes Cooking Time: 8 minutes Serve: 4

Ingredients:

- 1 cup broccoli, process into rice
- 3 cups cauliflower rice
- 1/4 cup mascarpone cheese
- 1/2 cup parmesan cheese, shredded
- 1/8 tsp ground cinnamon
- ¼ tsp garlic powder
- ¼ tsp onion powder
- 1/4 tsp pepper
- 1 tbsp butter, melted
- 1/2 tsp salt

Directions:

1. In a heat-safe bowl, mix together cauliflower, nutmeg, garlic powder, onion powder, butter, broccoli, pepper, and salt and microwave for 4 minutes.
2. Stir well and microwave for 2 minutes more.
3. Add cheese and microwave for 2 minutes.
4. Add mascarpone cheese and stir until it looks creamy.
5. Serve and enjoy.

Nutritional Value (Amount per Serving):

Calories 135

Fat 10 g

Carbohydrates 6 g

Sugar 2 g

Protein 8 g

Cholesterol 30 mg

SOUPS, STEWS & SALADS

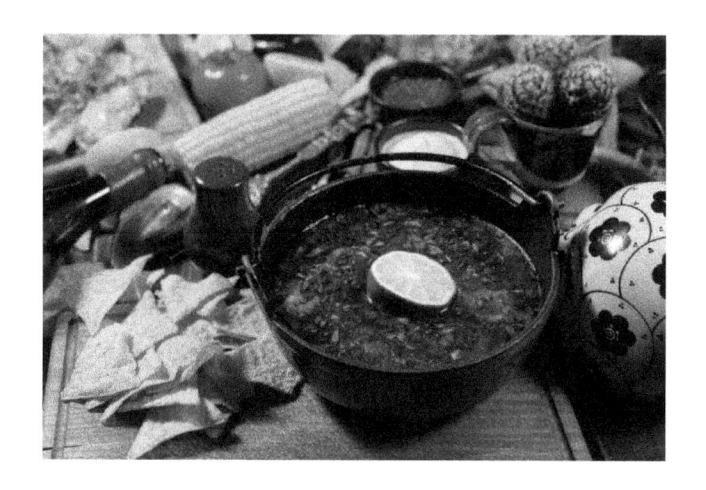

Hearty Cabbage Beef Soup

Preparation Time: 10 minutes Cooking Time: 45 minutes

Serve: 10

Ingredients:

- 2 lbs ground beef
- 4 cups chicken stock
- 10 oz Rotel tomatoes, diced
- 3 cube bouillon
- 1 large cabbage head, chopped
- ½ tsp cumin powder
- 2 garlic cloves, minced
- ¼ onion, diced
- Pepper
- Salt

Directions:

1. Brown the meat in pan over medium heat.
2. Add onion and cook until soften.
3. Transfer meat mixture to the stock pot.
4. Add remaining ingredients to the stock pot stir well and bring to boil over high heat.
5. Turn heat to medium-low and simmer for 45 minutes.

Nutritional Value (Amount per Serving):

Calories 260

Fat 18 g

Carbohydrates 5 g

Sugar 2 g

Protein 15 g

Cholesterol 64 mg

BRUNCH & DINNER

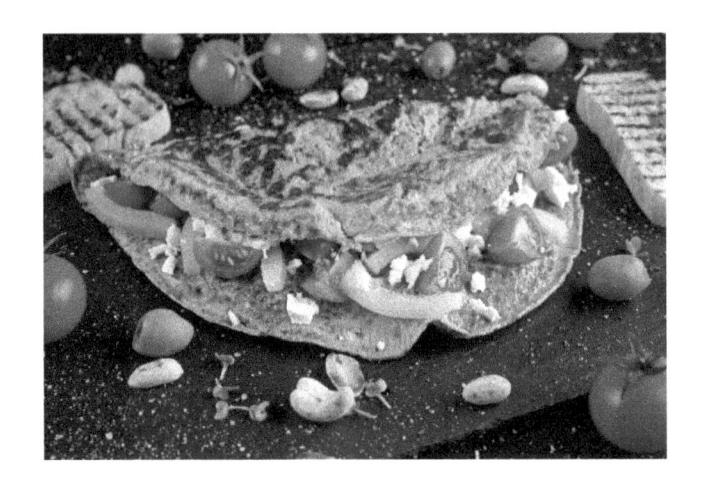

Cheese Almond Pancakes

Preparation Time: 10 minutes Cooking Time: 10 minutes Serve: 4

Ingredients:

- 4 eggs
- 1/4 tsp cinnamon
- 1/2 cup cream cheese
- 1/2 cup almond flour
- 1 tbsp butter, melted

Directions:

1. Add all ingredients into the blender and blend until combined.
2. Melt butter in a pan over medium heat.
3. Pour 3 tablespoons of batter per pancake and cook for 2 minutes on each side.
4. Serve and enjoy.

Nutritional Value (Amount per Serving):

Calories 271

Fat 25 g

Carbohydrates 5 g

Sugar 1 g

Protein 10.8 g

Cholesterol 203 mg

BREAKFAST RECIPES

Cauliflower Toast with Avocado

Serves: 2

Prep Time: 20 mins

Ingredients

- 1 large egg
- 1 small head cauliflower, grated
- 1 medium avocado, pitted and chopped
- ¾ cup mozzarella cheese, shredded
- Salt and black pepper, to taste

Directions

1. Preheat the oven to 420°F and line a baking sheet with parchment.
2. Place the cauliflower in a microwave safe bowl and microwave for about 7 minutes on high.
3. Spread on paper towels to drain after the cauliflower has completely cooled and press with a clean towel to remove excess moisture.
4. Put the cauliflower back in the bowl and stir in the mozzarella cheese and egg.
5. Season with salt and black pepper and stir until well combined.

6. Spoon the mixture onto the baking sheet in two rounded squares, as evenly as possible.
7. Bake for about 20 minutes until golden brown on the edges.
8. Mash the avocado with a pinch of salt and black pepper.
9. Spread the avocado onto the cauliflower toast and serve.

Nutrition Amount per serving

Calories 127 Total Fat 7g 9%

Saturated Fat 2.4g 12% Cholesterol 99mg 33%

Sodium 139mg 6%

Total Carbohydrate 9.1g 3% Dietary Fiber 4.8g 17% Total Sugars 3.4g

Protein 9.3g

DESSERTS & DRINKS

Cheesecake Fat Bombs

Preparation Time: 10 minutes Cooking Time: 10 minutes

Serve: 24

Ingredients:

- 8 oz cream cheese
- 1 ½ tsp vanilla
- 2 tbsp erythritol
- 4 oz coconut oil
- 4 oz heavy cream

Directions:

1. Add all ingredients into the mixing bowl and beat using immersion blender until creamy.
2. Pour batter into the mini cupcake liner and place in refrigerator until set.
3. Serve and enjoy.

Nutritional Value (Amount per Serving):

Calories 90

Fat 9.8 g

Carbohydrates 1.4 g

Sugar 0.1 g

Protein 0.8 g

Cholesterol 17 mg

APPETIZERS AND DESSERTS

Almond Flour Crackers

Serves: 6

Prep Time: 25 mins

Ingredients

- 2 tablespoons sunflower seeds
- 1 cup almond flour
- ¾ teaspoon sea salt
- 1 tablespoon whole psyllium husks
- 1 tablespoon coconut oil

Directions

1. Preheat the oven to 3500F and grease a baking sheet lightly.
2. Mix together sunflower seeds, almond flour, sea salt, coconut oil, psyllium husks and 2 tablespoons of water in a bowl.
3. Transfer into a blender and blend until smooth.
4. Form a dough out of this mixture and roll it on the parchment paper until 1/16 inch thick.
5. Slice into 1 inch squares and season with some sea salt.
6. Arrange the squares on the baking sheet and

transfer to the oven.
7. Bake for about 15 minutes until edges are crisp and brown.
8. Allow to cool and separate into squares to serve.

Nutrition Amount per serving

Calories 141

Total Fat 11.6g 15% Saturated Fat 2.7g 13%

Cholesterol 0mg 0%

Sodium 241mg 10%

Total Carbohydrate 5.2g 2% Dietary Fiber 3.1g

11% Total Sugars 0g

Protein 4.2g

PORK AND BEEF RECIPES

Cheesy Beef

Serves: 6

Prep Time: 40 mins

Ingredients

- 1 teaspoon garlic salt
- 2 pounds beef
- 1 cup cream cheese
- 1 cup mozzarella cheese, shredded
- 1 cup low carb Don Pablo's sauce

Directions

1. Season the meat with garlic salt and add to the instant pot.
2. Put the remaining ingredients in the pot and set the instant pot on low.
3. Cook for about 2 hours and dish out.

Nutrition Amount per serving

Calories 471

Total Fat 27.7g 36% Saturated Fat 14.6g 73%

Cholesterol 187mg 62%

Sodium 375mg 16%

Total Carbohydrate 2.9g 1% Dietary Fiber 0.1g 0%

Total Sugars 1.5g Protein 50.9g

Keto Minced Meat

Serves: 4

Prep Time: 30 mins

Ingredients

- 1 pound ground lamb meat
- 1 cup onions, chopped
- 2 tablespoons ginger garlic paste
- 3 tablespoons butter
- Salt and cayenne pepper, to taste

Directions

1. Put the butter in a pot and add garlic, ginger and onions.
2. Sauté for about 3 minutes and add ground meat and all the spices.
3. Cover the lid and cook for about 20 minutes on medium high heat.
4. Dish out to a large serving bowl and serve hot.

Nutrition Amount per serving

Calories 459

Total Fat 35.3g 45% Saturated Fat 14.7g 73%

Cholesterol 133mg 44%

Sodium 154mg 7%

Total Carbohydrate 4.8g 2% Dietary Fiber 0.6g 2%

Total Sugars 1.2g Protein 28.9g

Keto Taco Casserole

Serves: 8

Prep Time: 55 mins

Ingredients

- 2 pounds ground beef
- 1 tablespoon extra-virgin olive oil
- Taco seasoning mix, kosher salt and black pepper
- 2 cups Mexican cheese, shredded
- 6 large eggs, lightly beaten

Directions

1. Preheat the oven to 3600F and grease a 2 quart baking dish.
2. Heat oil over medium heat in a large skillet and add ground beef.
3. Season with taco seasoning mix, kosher salt and black pepper.
4. Cook for about 5 minutes on each side and dish out to let cool slightly.
5. Whisk together eggs in the beef mixture and transfer the mixture to the baking dish.
6. Top with Mexican cheese and bake for about 25 minutes until set.
7. Remove from the oven and serve warm.

Nutrition Amount per serving

Calories 382

Total Fat 21.6g 28% Saturated Fat 9.1g 45%

Cholesterol 266mg 89%

Sodium 363mg 16%

Total Carbohydrate 1.7g 1% Dietary Fiber 0g 0%

Total Sugars 0.4g Protein 45.3g

SEAFOOD RECIPES

Mahi Mahi Stew

Serves: 3

Prep Time: 45 mins

Ingredients

- 2 tablespoons butter
- 2 pounds Mahi Mahi fillets, cubed
- 1 onion, chopped
- Salt and black pepper, to taste
- 2 cups homemade fish broth

Directions

1. Season the Mahi Mahi fillets with salt and black pepper.
2. Heat butter in a pressure cooker and add onion.
3. Sauté for about 3 minutes and stir in the seasoned Mahi Mahi fillets and fish broth.
4. Lock the lid and cook on High Pressure for about 30 minutes.
5. Naturally release the pressure and dish out to serve hot.

Nutrition Amount per serving

Calories   398

Total Fat 12.5g 16% Saturated Fat 6.4g 32% Cholesterol 290mg 97%

Sodium 803mg 35%

Total Carbohydrate 5.5g 2% Dietary Fiber 1.5g 5%

Total Sugars 2.2g Protein 62.3g

VEGAN &
VEGETARIAN

Cauliflower Gratin

Serves: 6

Prep Time: 35 mins

Ingredients

- 20 oz. cauliflower, chopped
- 2 oz. salted butter, for frying
- 5 oz. cheddar cheese, shredded
- 15 oz. sausages in links, precooked and chopped into 1 inch pieces
- 1 cup crème fraiche

Directions

1. Preheat the oven to 3750F and grease a baking dish lightly.
2. Heat 1 oz. butter in a pan on medium low heat and add chopped cauliflower.
3. Sauté for about 4 minutes and transfer to the baking dish.
4. Heat the rest of the butter in a pan on medium low heat and add sausage links.
5. Sauté for about 3 minutes and transfer to the baking dish on top of cauliflower.
6. Pour the crème fraiche in the baking dish and top with

cheddar cheese.
7. Transfer into the oven and bake for about 15 minutes.
8. Dish out to a bowl and serve hot.

Nutrition Amount per serving

Calories 509

Total Fat 43.7g 56% Saturated Fat 21.3g 107%

Cholesterol 122mg 41%

Sodium 781mg 34%

Total Carbohydrate 7g 3% Dietary Fiber 2.4g 8%

Total Sugars 2.5g

Protein 22.8g

CHICKEN AND POULTRY RECIPES

Chicken Enchiladas

Serves: 2

Prep Time: 25 mins

Ingredients

- 2 ounces chicken, shredded
- ½ tablespoon olive oil
- 2 ounces shiitake mushrooms, chopped
- Sea salt and black pepper, to taste
- ½ teaspoon apple cider vinegar

Directions

1. Heat olive oil in a skillet and add mushrooms.
2. Sauté for about 30 seconds and stir in chicken.
3. Cook for about 2 minutes and pour in apple cider vinegar.
4. Season with sea salt and black pepper and cover the lid.
5. Cook for about 20 minutes on medium low heat.
6. Dish out and serve hot.

Nutrition Amount per serving

Calories 88

Total Fat 4.4g 6% Saturated Fat 0.8g 4%

Cholesterol 22mg 7%

Sodium 86mg 4%

Total Carbohydrate 3.9g 1% Dietary Fiber 0.6g 2%

Total Sugars 1g Protein 8.7g

BREAKFAST RECIPES

Cinnamon Noatmeal

Total Time: 10 minutes Serves: 2

Ingredients:

- ¾ cup hot water
- 2 tbsp sugar-free maple syrup
- ½ tsp ground cinnamon
- 2 tbsp ground flax seeds
- 3 tbsp vegan vanilla protein powder
- 3 tbsp hulled hemp seeds

Directions:

1. Add all ingredients into the bowl and stir until well combined.
2. Serve and enjoy.

Nutritional Value (Amount per Serving): Calories 220; Fat 12.5 g; Carbohydrates 9.5 g; Sugar 0.1 g; Protein 17.6 g; Cholesterol 0 mg;

Almond Coconut Porridge

Total Time: 10 minutes Serves: 2

Ingredients:

- ¾ cup unsweetened almond milk
- ½ tsp vanilla extract
- 1 ½ tbsp ground flaxseed
- 3 tbsp ground almonds
- 6 tbsp unsweetened shredded coconut
- Pinch of sea salt

Directions:

1. Add almond milk in microwave safe bowl and microwave for 2 minutes.
2. Add remaining ingredients and stir well and cook for 1 minute.
3. Top with fresh berries and serve.

Nutritional Value (Amount per Serving): Calories 197; Fat 17.4 g; Carbohydrates 8.3 g; Sugar 0.6 g; Protein 4.2 g; Cholesterol 0 mg;

Vegetable Tofu Scramble

Total Time: 20 minutes Serves: 2

Ingredients:

- 1 block firm tofu, drained and crumbled
- ½ tsp turmeric
- ¼ tsp garlic powder
- 1 cup spinach
- 1 red pepper, chopped
- 10 oz mushrooms, chopped
- ½ onion, chopped
- 1 tbsp olive oil
- Pepper
- Salt

Directions:

1. Heat olive oil in a large pan over medium heat.
2. Add onion, pepper, and mushrooms and sauté until cooked.

3. Add crumbled tofu, spices, and spinach. Stir well and cook for 3-5 minutes.
4. Serve and enjoy.

Nutritional Value (Amount per Serving): Calories 159; Fat 9.6 g; Carbohydrates 13.7 g; Sugar 7 g; Protein 9.6 g; Cholesterol 0 mg;

LUNCH RECIPES

Asparagus Mash

Total Time: 20 minutes Serves: 2

Ingredients:

- 10 asparagus shoots, chopped
- 1 tsp lemon juice
- 2 tbsp fresh parsley
- 2 tbsp coconut cream
- 1 small onion, diced
- 1 tbsp coconut oil
- Pepper
- Salt

Directions:

1. Sauté onion in coconut oil until onion is softened.
2. Blanch chopped asparagus in hot water for 2 minutes and drain immediately.
3. Add sautéed onion, lemon juice, parsley, coconut cream, asparagus, pepper, and salt into the blender and blend until smooth.
4. Serve warm and enjoy.

Nutritional Value (Amount per Serving): Calories 125; Fat 10.6 g; Carbohydrates 7.5 g; Sugar 3.6 g; Protein 2.6 g; Cholesterol 0 mg;

Classic Cabbage Slaw

Total Time: 20 minutes Serves: 3

Ingredients:

- 4 cups green cabbage, shredded
- 2 garlic cloves
- 1 tbsp sesame oil
- 2 tbsp tamari
- 1 tsp vinegar
- 1 tsp chili paste
- ½ cup macadamia nuts, chopped

Directions:

1. Toss shredded green cabbage in a pan with chili paste, sesame oil, vinegar, and tamari on medium-low heat.
2. Add garlic and cook for 5 minutes or until cabbage is softened.
3. Stir everything well. Add macadamia nuts and cook for 5 minutes.
4. Stir well and serve.

Nutritional Value (Amount per Serving): Calories 240; Fat 21.8 g; Carbohydrates 10.5 g; Sugar 4.7 g; Protein 4.5 g; Cholesterol 1 mg;

Delicious Herb Cauliflower Rice

Total Time: 20 minutes Serves: 3

Ingredients:

- 10 oz cauliflower rice
- 4 oz mushrooms, sliced
- 8 oz asparagus, cut into 3" pieces
- 1/2 tsp rosemary
- 1/2 tsp cayenne
- 2 tbsp olive oil
- 6 baby carrots, sliced
- 1/2 tsp black pepper
- 1/2 tsp sea salt

Directions:

1. Heat olive oil in a pan over medium heat.
2. Add vegetables to a pan and sauté for 3-4 minutes.
3. Add cauliflower rice and spices and sauté for 10 minutes.
4. Serve and enjoy.

Nutritional Value (Amount per Serving): Calories 137; Fat 9.7 g; Carbohydrates 11.5 g; Sugar 5.3 g; Protein 5 g; Cholesterol 0 mg; ;

DINNER RECIPES

Almond Green Beans

Total Time: 20 minutes Serves: 4

Ingredients:

- 1 lb fresh green beans, trimmed
- 1/3 cup almonds, sliced
- 4 garlic cloves, sliced
- 2 tbsp olive oil
- 1 tbsp lemon juice
- ½ tsp sea salt

Directions:

1. Add green beans, salt, and lemon juice in a mixing bowl. Toss well and set aside.
2. Heat oil in a pan over medium heat.
3. Add sliced almonds and sauté until lightly browned.
4. Add garlic and sauté for 30 seconds.
5. Pour almond mixture over green beans and toss well.
6. Stir well and serve immediately.

Nutritional Value (Amount per Serving): Calories 146; Fat 11.2 g; Carbohydrates 10.9 g; Sugar 2 g; Protein 4 g; Cholesterol 0 mg;

Fried Okra

Total Time: 20 minutes Serves: 4

Ingredients:

- 1 lb fresh okra, cut into ¼" slices
- 1/3 cup almond meal
- Pepper
- Salt
- Oil for frying

Directions:

1. Heat oil in large pan over medium- high heat.
2. In a bowl, mix together sliced okra, almond meal, pepper, and salt until well coated.
3. Once the oil is hot then add okra to the hot oil and cook until lightly browned.
4. Remove fried okra from pan and allow to drain on paper towels.
5. Serve and enjoy.

Nutritional Value (Amount per Serving): Calories 91; Fat 4.2 g; Carbohydrates 10.2 g; Sugar 10.2 g; Protein 3.9 g; Cholesterol 0 mg;

DESSERT RECIPES

Lemon Mousse

Total Time: 10 minutes Serves: 2

Ingredients:

- 14 oz coconut milk
- 12 drops liquid stevia
- 1/2 tsp lemon extract
- 1/4 tsp turmeric

Directions:

1. Place coconut milk can in the refrigerator for overnight. Scoop out thick cream into a mixing bowl.
2. Add remaining ingredients to the bowl and whip using a hand mixer until smooth.
3. Transfer mousse mixture to a zip-lock bag and pipe into small serving glasses. Place in refrigerator.
4. Serve chilled and enjoy.

Nutritional Value (Amount per Serving): Calories 444; Fat 45.7 g; Carbohydrates 10 g; Sugar 6 g; Protein 4.4 g; Cholesterol 0 mg;

BREAKFAST RECIPES

Burrito Bowl

This is a burrito that does not even need the tortillas to deliver this nourishing low carb breakfast.

Total Prep & Cooking Time: 30 minutes Level: Intermediate

Makes: 12 Fat Bombs Protein: 14 grams

Net Carbs: 4 grams Fat: 14 grams

Sugar: 2 grams

Calories: 299

What you need:

- 1/2 lb. ground beef, lean
- 3/4 cup water
- 1 cup cauliflower
- 2 tbs cilantro, chopped
- 1 tsp butter, melted
- 3 large eggs
- 1/4 tsp salt
- 3 tsp taco seasoning
- 1/8 tsp pepper

Steps:

1. Split the cauliflower into pieces and place in a food blender. Pulse for approximately 60 seconds until crumbly.

2. Heat the cauliflower in a saucepan for about 5 minutes as it becomes tender. Remove from heat.
3. Spoon the cauliflower into a tea towel and wring to eliminate the excess water. Repeat this step as many times as necessary to ensure the liquid has been removed. Put aside.
4. In another dish, beat the eggs and butter together and set to the side.
5. Use a skillet to brown the ground beef for approximately 7 minutes. Drain the fat and stir the water and taco seasoning into the meat.
6. Boil the water and reduce the heat. Allow to rest for approximately 3 additional minutes while simmering.
7. Section off the meat to one side of the pan. Pour the riced cauliflower into the clear area of the pan and sprinkle with the cilantro.
8. Heat and brown for approximately 4 minutes and press to the side of the pan to clear space for the egg mixture.
9. Prepare the eggs to your preference and then combine everything in the pan fully.
10. Spice with the seasons to your personal taste and serve.

Baking Tip:

If you find that your skillet is not large enough to cook all the ingredients in one pan, use a separate frying pan as necessary.

LUNCH RECIPES

Burger Cabbage Stir Fry

This quick lunch dish is easy to whip up even in the morning so it can be brought with you to work.

Total Prep & Cooking Time: 20 minutes

Level: Beginner Makes: 4 Helpings

Protein: 9 grams Net Carbs: 1.5 grams Fat: 8 grams

Sugar: 1 gram

Calories: 208

What you need:

- 1/4 tsp salt
- 5 oz. ground beef
- 1 tsp onion powder
- 8 oz. cabbage, sliced
- 1 clove garlic, minced
- 2 tbs coconut oil
- 1/8 tsp pepper

Steps:

1. In a big skillet, combine the bacon and beef and brown for approximately 7 minutes.
2. Then fry the minced garlic, chopped cabbage and onion powder with the meat for about 2 additional minutes.
3. Serve warm after seasoning with pepper and salt.

Baking Tip:

For this stir fry, you can also use a wok instead of the skillet.

UNUSUAL DELICIOUS MEAL RECIPES

Calamari Salad

This meal might look a little bit too unusual, but it will build your muscles after that powerful workout.

Total Prep & Cooking Time: 10 minutes Level: Beginner

Makes: 4 Helpings

Protein: 18 grams Net Carbs: 5 grams

Fat: 14 grams

Sugar: 0 grams

Calories: 214

What you need:

- 1/2 tsp lime juice
- 16 oz. calamari, sliced
- 1/4 tsp salt
- 2 tbs coconut oil
- 1/8 tsp pepper
- 8 oz. olives
- 1/2 tsp garlic powder
- 3 tsp coconut oil, separate
- 1/2 tsp lemon juice

Steps:
1. In a glass dish, blend the lemon and lime juice fully.
2. In a separate dish, whisk the 3 teaspoons of coconut oil, salt, garlic powder, and pepper until combined.
3. In a non-stick skillet, dissolve the 2 tablespoons of coconut oil with the olives. Heat the olives for about 90 seconds and remove to a serving plate.
4. Coat the calamari liberally in the seasonings.
5. Transfer the calamari to the hot oil and stir fry for approximately 2 minutes or until they become cloudy.
6. Remove to the serving plate with the olives.
7. Drizzle the juice dressing over the top of the plate and serve.

KETO DESSERTS RECIPES

Coconut Lemon Bars

Serves: 24

Preparation time: 10 minutes Cooking time: 42 minutes

Ingredients:

- 4 eggs
- 1 tbsp coconut flour
- 3/4 cup Swerve
- 1/2 tsp baking powder
- 1/3 cup fresh lemon juice
- For crust:
- 1/4 cup Swerve
- 2 1/4 cups almond flour
- 1/2 cup coconut oil, melted

Directions:

1. Preheat the oven to 350 F/ 180 C.
2. Spray a baking dish with cooking spray and set aside.
3. In a small bowl, mix together 1/4 cup swerve and almond flour.
4. Add melted coconut oil and mix until it forms into a dough.

5. Transfer dough into the prepared pan and spread evenly.
6. Bake for 15 minutes.
7. For the filling: Add eggs, coconut flour, baking powder, lemon juice, and swerve into the blender and blend for 10 seconds.
8. Pour blended mixture on top of baked crust and spread well.
9. Bake for 25 minutes.
10. Remove from oven and set aside to cool completely.
11. Slice and serve.

Per Serving: Net Carbs: 1.5g; Calories: 113; Total Fat: 10.6g; Saturated Fat: 4.6g

Protein: 3.3g; Carbs: 2.8g; Fiber: 1.3g; Sugar: 0.5g; Fat 84% / Protein 11% / Carbs 5%

CAKE

Fudgy Chocolate Cake

Serves: 12

Preparation time: 10 minutes Cooking time: 30 minutes

Ingredients:

- 6 eggs
- 1 ½ cup erythritol
- ½ cup almond flour
- oz butter, melted
- oz unsweetened chocolate, melted
- Pinch of salt

Directions:

1. Preheat the oven to 350 F/ 180 C.
2. Grease 8-inch spring-form cake pan with butter and set aside.
3. In a large bowl, beat eggs until foamy.
4. Add sweetener and stir well.
5. Add melted butter, chocolate, almond flour, and salt and stir until combined.
6. Pour batter in the prepared cake pan and bake in preheated oven for 30 minutes.
7. Remove cake from oven and allow to cool completely.
8. Slice and serve.

Per Serving: Net Carbs: 4g; Calories: 360; Total Fat: 37.6g; Saturated Fat: 21.6g

Protein: 7.2g; Carbs: 8.6g; Fiber: 4.6g; Sugar: 0.6g; Fat 90% / Protein 7% / Carbs 3%

Coconut Cake

Serves: 8

Preparation time: 10 minutes Cooking time: 20 minutes

Ingredients:

- 5 eggs, separated
- ½ tsp baking powder
- ½ tsp vanilla
- ½ cup butter softened
- ½ cup erythritol
- ¼ cup unsweetened coconut milk
- ½ cup coconut flour
- Pinch of salt

Directions:

1. Preheat the oven to 400 F/ 200 C.
2. Grease cake pan with butter and set aside.
3. In a bowl, beat sweetener and butter until combined.
4. Add egg yolks, coconut milk, and vanilla and mix well.
5. Add baking powder, coconut flour, and salt and stir well.
6. In another bowl, beat egg whites until stiff peak forms.
7. Gently fold egg whites into the cake mixture.
8. Pour batter in a prepared cake pan and bake in preheated oven for 20 minutes.

9. Slice and serve.

Per Serving: Net Carbs: 0.8g; Calories: 163 Total Fat: 16.2g; Saturated Fat: 9.9g

Protein: 3.9g; Carbs: 1.3g; Fiber: 0.5g; Sugar: 0.6g; Fat 89% / Protein 9% / Carbs 2%

Intermediate:
Lemon Cake

Serves: 10

Preparation time: 10 minutes Cooking time: 60 minutes

Ingredients:

- 4 eggs
- 2 tbsp lemon zest
- ½ cup fresh lemon juice
- ¼ cup erythritol
- 1 tbsp vanilla
- ½ cup butter softened
- 2 tsp baking powder
- ¼ cup coconut flour
- 2 cups almond flour

Directions:

1. Preheat the oven to 300 F/ 150 C.
2. Grease 9-inch loaf pan with butter and set aside.
3. In a large bowl, whisk all ingredients until a smooth batter is formed.
4. Pour batter into the loaf pan and bake in preheated oven for 60 minutes.
5. Slice and serve.

Per Serving: Net Carbs: 3.6g; Calories: 244; Total Fat: 22.3g; Saturated Fat: 7.3g Protein: 7.3g; Carbs: 6.3g; Fiber: 2.7g; Sugar: 1.5g; Fat 83% / Protein 12% / Carbs 5%

Tarts and Pie:
Beginner

Peanut Butter Pie Serves: 16

Preparation time: 15 minutes Cooking time: 10 minutes

Ingredients:

For crust:

- ¾ cup almond flour
- ½ cup of cocoa powder
- ½ cup erythritol
- 1/3 cup almond butter
- ½ cup butter softened

For filling:

- 1 ½ cups heavy whipping cream
- ½ cup erythritol
- 1/3 cup peanut butter
- 8 oz cream cheese, softened

Directions:

1. For the crust: In a large bowl, combine together butter, cocoa powder, sweetener, and almond butter until smooth.
2. Add almond flour and beat until mixture stiff.
3. Transfer crust mixture into the greased spring-form cake pan and spread evenly and place in the

refrigerator for 15-30 minutes.
4. Meanwhile for filling: In a mixing bowl, beat sweetener, peanut butter, and cream cheese until smooth.
5. Add heavy cream and beat until stiff peaks form.
6. Spread filling mixture in prepared crust and refrigerate for 2 hours.
7. Slice and serve.

Per Serving: Net Carbs: 2.7g; Calories: 209;

Total Fat: 20.7g; Saturated Fat: 10.3g

Protein: 4.4g; Carbs: 4.4g; Fiber: 1.7g; Sugar: 0.8g; Fat 88% / Protein 7% / Carbs 5%

FROZEN DESSERT: BEGINNER

Raspberry Sorbet

Serves: 5

Preparation time: 10 minutes Cooking time: 10 minutes

Ingredients:

- 2 1/2 cups fresh raspberries
- 1 tbsp fresh lemon juice
- 1/3 cup erythritol
- 1/3 cup unsweetened coconut milk
- 1 tsp liquid stevia
- Pinch of sea salt

Directions:

1. Add all ingredients into the blender and blend until smooth.
2. Transfer blended mixture into the container and place in the refrigerator for 20 minutes.
3. After 20 minutes pour sorbet mixture into the ice cream maker and churn according to the machine instructions.
4. Pour into the air-tight container and place in the refrigerator for 1-2 hours.
5. Serve chilled and enjoy.

Per Serving: Net Carbs: 4g; Calories: 41; Total Fat: 1.9g; Saturated Fat: 0.7g

Protein: 1g; Carbs: 8g; Fiber: 4g; Sugar: 2.8g; Fat 45% / Protein 10% / Carbs 45%

BREAKFAST RECIPES

Broken Black Pepper Bread

Complete: 4 hr 45 min

Prep: 4 hr

Cook: 45 min

Yield: 1 portion bread

Nutritional Values:

Calories: 34, Total Fat: 5.1 g, Saturated Fat: 0.3 g, Carbs: 1.5 g, Sugars: 0.3 g, Protein: 1.3 g

Ingredients

- 2 cups in addition to 2 tablespoons milk
- 3 tablespoons unsalted spread
- 2 tablespoons sugar
- 1/2 teaspoons butcher's crush broke dark pepper
- One 1/4-ounce bundle dynamic dry yeast
- 5 cups generally useful flour
- 1 tablespoon fine salt
- Vegetable oil, as required

Direction

1. In a little pot, consolidate the milk, spread, sugar, and pepper. Spot over medium-high warmth and achieve to

110 degrees F. Expel from the warmth and sprinkle the yeast over the outside of the milk. Put aside until frothy, around 10 minutes.

2. In the mean time, in an enormous bowl, whisk together the flour and salt.

3. Pour the milk and yeast blend into the bowl of flour and blend until a delicate, battered blend is shaped. Move the blend to a well-floured work surface and ply until a delicate versatile batter is framed, around 10 minutes. Move the mixture to a softly oiled bowl, spread with a kitchen towel, and spot in a warm spot, until puffed and multiplied in size, around 2 hours.

4. Spot a rack in the focal point of the broiler and preheat to 400 degrees F. Move the mixture to the work surface and, utilizing your hands, delicately straighten it into a 10-inch-long oval shape. Crease the batter into thirds longwise, covering the sides in the inside. Press down on the covering sides to seal and make a crease. Spot it crease side-down in a buttered 9 by 5- inch portion dish, spread with a kitchen towel, and come back to the hottest piece of the kitchen until the mixture has ascended around 1/2 crawls over the highest point of the container, around 1/2 to 2 hours.

5. Brush the highest point of the batter gently with warm water and, utilizing a sharp blade, make 1/4-inch-profound cut down the middle. Prepare until brilliant darker, around 30 minutes.

6. Expel the portion from the skillet and spot in the focal

point of the rack. Keep heating until the portion sounds empty when riveted gently with your knuckles on the base and top, and a thermometer embedded in the inside peruses 200 degrees F., around 15 minutes.

7. Move the bread portion to a cooling rack and let cool for 2 hours before utilizing.

LUNCH RECIPES

Herb Bread

Nutritional Values:

Calories: 421, Total Fat: 37.4 g, Saturated Fat: 14.8 g, Carbs: 9.4 g, Sugars: 0.9 g, Protein: 15.1 g Serves: 4

Ingredients:

- 2 Tbsp Coconut Flour
- 1 ½ cups Almond Flour
- 2 Tbsp Fresh Herbs of choice, chopped
- 2 Tbsp Ground Flax Seeds
- 1 ½ tsp Baking Soda
- ¼ tsp Salt
- 5 Eggs
- 1 Tbsp Apple Cider Vinegar
- ¼ cup Coconut Oil, melted

Directions:

1. Preheat your oven to 350F / 175C. Grease a loaf pan and set aside.
2. Add the coconut flour, almond flour, herbs, flax, baking soda, and salt to your food processor. Pulse to combine and then add the eggs, vinegar, and oil.

3. Transfer the batter to the prepared loaf pan and bake in the preheated oven for about half an hour.
4. Once baked and golden brown, remove from the oven, set aside to cool, slice and eat.

Spicy Cloud Bread

Cooking time: 25-30 min Yield: 6 clouds

Nutrition facts: 52 calories per cloud: Carbs 2.8g, fats 3.4g, and proteins 3.1g.

Ingredients:

- 3 eggs
- 4 tbsp xylitol
- 2 tbsp cream cheese
- 2 tsp cinnamon, ground
- ½ tsp baking powder
- vanilla to taste

Steps:

1. Heat the oven to 175 C.
2. Prepare the baking sheet.
3. Beat the egg whites with baking powder for 2-3 min using a hand mixer until stiff peaks.
4. Mix yolks+cream cheese+vanilla+xylitol+cinnamon.
5. Combine whites with yolks softly.
6. Form 6 mounds and place the dough onto the baking sheet, greased. Make them flat.
7. Bake for 30 min until they are golden.

SNACKS RECIPES

Sesame bread

Servings: 3

Cooking time: 20 minutes

Nutrients per one serving:

Calories: 82 | Fats: 12 g | Carbs: 1 g | Proteins: 7 g

Ingredients:

- 5 tbsp sesame flour
- 1 egg
- 1 tbsp butter
- ½ tsp baking powder
- A pinch of salt

Cooking process:

1. Mix the ingredients.
2. Melt the butter to room temperature.

Add butter and egg to the mass, mix well.

3. Pour the dough into a baking dish and bake in the oven at 180°C (356°F) for 15 minutes.

Buns with sesame

Servings: 4

Cooking time: 50 minutes

Nutrients per one serving: Calories: 95 | Fats: 10 g | Carbs: 5 g | Proteins: 13.1 g

Ingredients for the dough:
- ¾ cup almond flour
- 1 egg
- oz mozzarella
- 2 tbsp cream cheese
- 1 tsp stevia

Ingredients for sprinkling:
- 1 tbsp butter
- 1 tbsp sesame seeds

Cooking process:
1. The oven to be preheated to 200°C (400°F).
2. In a bowl, mix the flour, stevia, and egg. Leave mass for 5 minutes.
3. In the microwave oven, melt the cream cheese. Add chopped mozzarella, mix until uniformity. Add the cheese mass to the flour and mix again. Knead a dough. Divide the dough into 4 pieces, form rings from the dough.
4. Cover the baking sheet with parchment, and lay out the buns. Grease buns with melted butter and sprinkle with sesame.

5. Bake in the oven for 20 minutes. Lay out them onto a plate and cool down.

THE KETO LUNCH

Tuesday: Lunch:

Mason Jar Salad

So colorful and full of flavor. This salad is portable. Use any vegetable you have on hand.

Variation tip: try different kinds of protein, cheese or seeds.

Prep Time: 10 minutes Cook Time: None

Servings: 1

What's in it

- Cooked, diced chicken (4 ounces)
- Baby spinach (1/6 ounce)
- Cherry tomatoes (1/6 ounce)
- Bell pepper (1/6 ounce)
- Cucumber (1/6 ounce)
- Green onion (1/2 qty)
- Extra virgin olive oil (4 T)

How it's made
1. Chop vegetables.
2. Stuff spinach at the bottom of jar.
3. Layer the rest of the vegetables.
4. Keep olive oil in a separate container until ready to eat.

Net carbs: 4 grams Fat: 55 grams

Protein: 71 grams

Sugars: 1 gram

Wednesday: Lunch: The Smoked Salmon Special

This may be the easiest lunch special ever.

Flavorful, smoky, pink salmon poses on your plate next to dark, green spinach as a feast for the eyes and the body.

Variation tip: serve with arugula or cabbage. Prep Time: 5 minutes Cook Time: None Serves 2

What's in it

- Wild caught smoked salmon (.5 ounces)
- Mayonnaise (generous dollop)
- Baby spinach (large handful)
- Extra virgin olive oil (.5 T)
- Lime wedge (1 qty)
- Kosher salt (to taste)
- Fresh ground pepper (to taste)

How it's made

1. Place salmon (or any fatty fish like sardines or mackerel) and spinach on a plate.
2. Add a large spoonful of mayonnaise and the lime wedge.
3. Drizzle oil atop the baby spinach (or try arugula or cabbage shredded as if for slaw)
4. Sprinkle with a little salt and pepper. Net carbs: None

Fat: 109 gramsProtein: 105 grams Sugars: None

KETO AT DINNER

Thursday: Dinner: On the go chicken wings with green beans

We decided to incorporate a meal idea here to illustrate how you can build your keto meals when you're pressed for time.

What's In it:

- Pecan smoked chicken wings (frozen, available at WalMart)
- Marketside French Green beans (fresh and packaged for microwaving, available at Walmart.
- How it's made:
- Preheat oven to 425.
- Bake chicken wings for 30-35 minutes.
- When chicken wings are almost done, place beans inside a microwave in the bag and cook for 2-3 minutes.
- Take beans out and season with butter or olive oil, and salt and pepper.

- Enjoy with your chicken wings!

Net carbs: 7 grams

1. Fat: 14 grams per 4 ounces serving of chicken, be sure to add butter or olive oil used
2. Protein: 14 grams per 4 ounces serving of chicken
3. Sugars: 3 grams

CPSIA information can be obtained
at www.ICGtesting.com
Printed in the USA
LVHW050955220221
679615LV00003B/551